The Little
Book of
Ayurveda

In memory of Wallace, the best cat in the world, who helped immeasurably with the work that led to this book.

The Little
Book of
Ayurveda

Ignacja Glebe

An Hachette UK Company
www.hachette.co.uk

First published in Great Britain in 2021 by Gaia, an imprint of
Octopus Publishing Group Ltd
Carmelite House
50 Victoria Embankment
London EC4Y 0DZ
www.octopusbooks.co.uk

Text copyright © Octopus Publishing Group Limited 2021

Distributed in the US by Hachette Book Group
1290 Avenue of the Americas
4th and 5th Floors
New York, NY 10104

Distributed in Canada by
Canadian Manda Group
664 Annette St.
Toronto, Ontario,
Canada M6S 2C8

ISBN 978-1-85675-440-8

A CIP catalogue record for this book is available from the British Library.

Printed and bound in China
10 9 8 7 6 5 4 3 2 1

All reasonable care has been taken in the preparation of this book but the information it
contains is not intended to take the place of treatment by a qualified medical practitioner.
Before making any changes in your health regime, always consult a doctor. While the
cleanse detailed in this book is completely safe if done correctly, you must seek professional
advice if you are in any doubt about any medical condition. Any application of the ideas
and information contained in this book is at the reader's sole discretion and risk.

Commissioning Editor: Natalie Bradley
Editorial Assistant: Sarah Kyle
Art Director: Juliette Norsworthy
Production Manager: Allison Gonsalves
Copy Editor: Clare Churly
Proofreader: Tara O'Sullivan
Design and illustration: Abi Read

Contents

Introduction: Balance

This is a book about an ancient system of wisdom; a book about medicine and energy and the way we live; a book about how we eat, how we sleep, how we move and even how we breathe; a book that touches on every element of our lives. But that seems like a lot for the first page, doesn't it? Let's say, for now, simply: this is a book about balance.

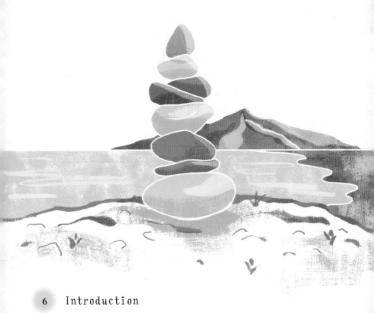

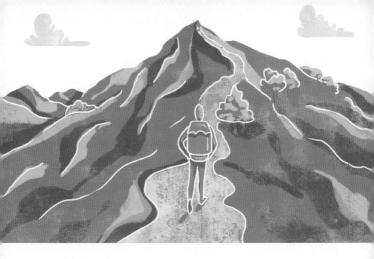

It's difficult, these days, not to feel a little askew sometimes. I know. I get it. I feel it, and you do, too, right? We all do. The world goes so fast, and it can be hard not to feel like you're falling behind. Your to-do list (if it's anything like mine) goes on for miles – and you could write another one just as long for tomorrow.

Sometimes it seems like you've started climbing a mountain without knowing what's at the summit, or even asking yourself whether you really wanted to climb it at all. You've got so much on, and so many demands on your limited time – and yet, somehow, here you are. Here we are together, in a moment we've taken back from everyone else, and given purely and simply to ourselves.

By reading the first pages of this book, designed specifically to bring better balance into your life, you've taken the first step toward becoming your best, balanced self: you've tipped the scale just a little further in your favour than it was when you woke up this morning.

In this little book, we'll run through a series of exercises, quizzes and ideas designed to push your body and mind back into gear. These ideas are all taken from Ayurveda, the ancient Indian science of life. In fact, "the science of life" is the literal

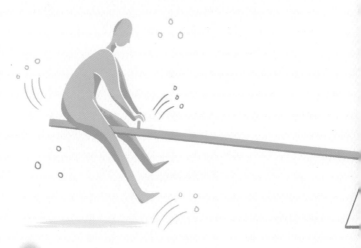

meaning of the Sanskrit word *Ayurveda*. So what does this ancient system of wisdom have to offer us in the modern world? What can something first imagined before the pyramids were constructed, before horses were tamed, and before numbers were invented have to tell us about life in the 21st century?

The thing is: times change, but people don't. Not really. We want and need the same things we've always wanted and needed; we're made of the same basic stuff as our ancestors; we're fashioned after the same pattern. It's just that modern life gets in the way, making it hard to see how simple we really are, and what is it that we really need.

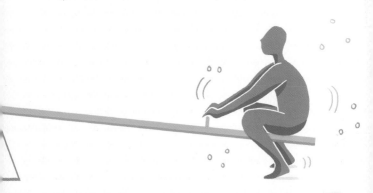

Maslow's Hierarchy of Needs

Some five thousand years after the gurus of Ayurveda first began their work, a psychologist named Abraham Maslow developed a theory called the hierarchy of needs. Perhaps you have heard of it. It looks like this:

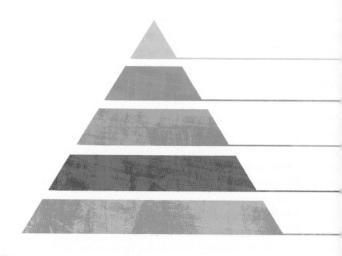

This pyramid – although it's important to say right away that later theories have talked about it less as a pyramid, and more as a series of overlapping desires – represents the things humans need. (Actually, until you reach the top tier, it represents those things that most animals need, too.) We need to eat, to sleep, to move, to breathe. We need to feel safe, and to know that we can eat and sleep and breathe in safety. We need each other, and we need space within and from and around one another to become the best we can be.

Self-actualization
Desire to become the most that one can be.

Esteem
Respect, self-esteem, status, recognition, strength, freedom.

Love and belonging
Friendship, intimacy, family, sense of connection.

Safety needs
Personal security, employment, resources, health, property.

Physiological needs
Air, water, food, shelter, sleep, clothing, reproduction.

EXERCISE:

Examine Your Needs

Before we go any further, let's consider how many of these needs are currently being met in your life. You'll need to grab some paper and a pen for this exercise.

1 Sketch out a blank five-tiered pyramid, copying the illustration on page 10.

2 For each tier, consider the needs that Maslow outlined and then write down anything that's a stress, or a want, or that's lacking in your life. Are there things you wish for and don't have, or don't have enough of? Are you hungry, tired or touch-starved? Are you worried about your job or your relationships?

3 Now look at where your needs are clustered. Are they higher up the pyramid or are they lower down? Are there needs you could meet right away, and if not, why not? What's getting in the way?

4 Look particularly hard at any unmet needs higher up the pyramid. Ask yourself whether they could be brought lower. If you feel you're lacking in self-esteem, for example, is that because your job is unfulfilling? And are you in that unfulfilling job because you don't have the energy to find another one? And is that because you're tired? How's your sleep? How's your diet? How many of your higher-level wants and needs are being held back by a lack of balance in these most basic requirements? (More than you'd think at first, I'll bet.)

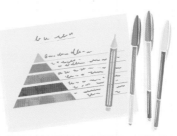

Better Balance

The desires we have now, in the 21st century, aren't new. They didn't spring into being when Maslow drew up his hierarchy of needs in the 1940s. They are mostly very basic — and very ancient. We're the latest in a long line of soft animals who want these things, and because we are so young, there's much we can learn from the millennia of wisdom that came before us.

We're going to use Ayurveda, the ancient science of life, to satisfy our unmet desires, and to shore up those we believe we've already solved. Ayurveda is a holistic tradition that, at its heart, takes the most basic tier of

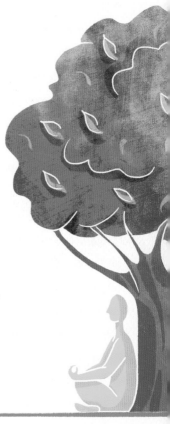

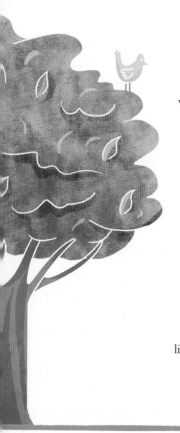

Maslow's needs and transforms it into a world view through which we can achieve anything else we want. It's a tradition stretching back more than five thousand years, and yet one that can work in tandem with modern science, too.

There are many benefits to the Ayurvedic lifestyle that Western science is only just discovering, which is old news to the millions around the globe who've made Ayurvedic practice into a way of life. In this book, you'll learn to incorporate Ayurvedic ways, little by little, into your own life. These ways amount, very simply, to better balance.

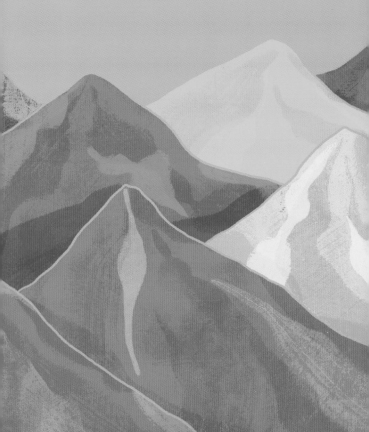

1. *Dosha*

Holistic Healing

The body, mind and consciousness are united; to treat one is to treat the others, too. You can't separate them out into their constituent parts. You can't expect one to recover while ignoring the others, and you can't have symptoms in one without experiencing trouble in the others, too. Things go together. The body is a whole.

This concept is starting to become clear to even the most cynical of Western medics. Think about how our mental and physical health is almost always linked. Chronic physical illness is often associated with a rise in depression and anxiety, and we are starting to see that we can sometimes alleviate the symptoms of mental illness by making physical changes to diet or exercise regimes.

It's clear that the mental health benefits of eating well, sleeping well and exercising cannot be overstated – and yet they're so often ignored in favour of prescribed medicine. We must consider the root cause and go back to those basic needs. Are they being met? If so, are they being met correctly? And are they being met correctly for us?

Every Person is Unique

Unlike Western medicine, Ayurveda takes as its starting point the concept that not all bodies are the same. Not all bodies are the same; not all minds are the same; not all personalities are the same. Our personalities are formed by our experiences of living in our own bodies and with our own minds. Each of us is the product of the life we have lived, shaped irrevocably by our bodies and brains. The way we think is changed by the things we have done and the things that are done to us; the things we do are shaped by the things we think, which are formed, in turn, by both nature and nurture.

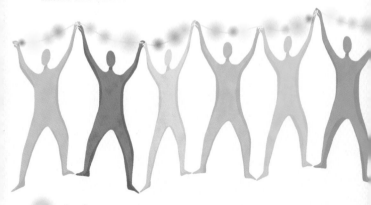

When we look at it like this, it seems crazy to accept a system that could treat an illness of the body without considering the effect on the mind, or to treat a mental illness without considering the fundamental differences between the way two different people might react to the same interventions. The way I respond to feeling blue won't be the same as the way you respond. We might need different help, and different support. Mind, body and consciousness are inextricably linked, and the ways in which they are linked are not the same for everybody.

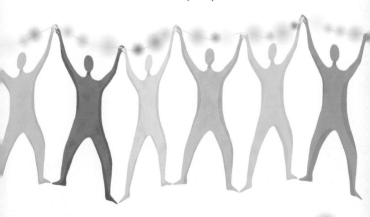

We Are All Built Differently

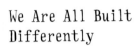

This seems self-explanatory, right? It seems so obvious, in fact, that you don't even know why I'm taking the time to tell you about it.

Well, I agree. However, in the West we have this idea of the perfect body. It's the body to which all people, given sufficient "self-control", should aspire. You know this body: it's in every diet book, exercise manual and glossy magazine.

Every diet promises to give you this body; every exercise regime promises to help you keep it; and every glossy magazine promises that, once you have that body, you'll want for nothing ever again. Everything is predicated on the possibility of every person being able to reduce themselves (or grow themselves) into one particular kind of body, and it's simply not true.

We pretend, in the West, that our bodies all need the same things from food, or sleep, or exercise. We pretend that a diet is a one-size-fits-all solution (pun intended). We think that "calories in, calories out" works for everyone, and, indeed, that it "works" to achieve something desirable. We assume that the perfect body is the ultimate goal – but this simply isn't true. It's not achievable. Diet culture, as far as changing your body physically is concerned, is a scam.

Bodies simply aren't meant to lose weight in the way modern diets promise: it's not evolutionarily useful to your body to lose weight for no reason. Weight loss through dieting is extremely unlikely – and it's also unlikely to lead to significant changes in health outcomes. Many studies show that most dieters (between 60 and 95 per cent) revert to their original body type after six months. Furthermore, it's not just pointless: it's also harmful. Diet culture not only damages our relationships to food, eating and living, it also physically alters our metabolisms, making them less efficient.

Assuming that all bodies are built the same, and run the same, is dangerous. Which brings us back to Ayurveda, a tradition that acknowledges at its heart that there is more than one body type, and that people are different, and built differently. Ayurveda acknowledges that people bring different qualities to the table, according to their abilities, and require different things from it, according to their needs.

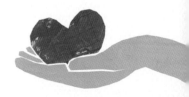

The *Doshas*

Ayurvedic medicine considers there to be three main body types (personality types and consciousness types). These body types are called *doshas,* and knowing your *dosha* can help you work out what to eat, how to move, how to sleep, how to breathe and how to take care of yourself.

pitta

The three main *doshas* are called *pitta, vata* and *kapha.* Most people have one dominant *dosha,* some have two, and some very rare people have all three in equal measure. Your *dosha* serves as your *prakriti:* your natural state, how you were meant to be. You don't need to change this natural state. You don't need to be something you're not. You just need to work out how best to work with what you were given, how best to care for what you have, and how to only take from the world what you need to balance yourself out. It's about being the best *you* you can possibly be.

vata

kapha

We can't change who we are and we shouldn't try to. But in order to be happy and healthy, we need to work with our natural state to achieve a sense of equilibrium. We need to have a balance of all three *doshas*. We need *pitta, vata* and *kapha* (fire, air and earth) in harmony within us to keep us grounded and together. They are influenced by what we eat, what we do, how we move, how we breathe and where we are.

The important thing to note right now is that we're in charge of these *doshas*. They are within our control, and we can find our truest selves – our *prakriti* – starting right now. Like increases like, and opposites balance opposites. If you're slow and heavy by nature, do exercises that make you feel light and fast. If you're agitated and unfocused by nature, live in a way that makes you feel more grounded. It's obvious, right? Your current state – how you are right now – is called your *vikriti*. Problems in life arise when your *vikriti* and *prakriti* aren't aligned – when who you're trying to be is fighting against who you are, and when your wants are contradictory to your needs.

Think of it kind of like something from Zen Buddhism: suffering isn't caused by the world, but by our desire to change the world so that it conforms to some idea we've invented of how it ought to be. Suffering in the Ayurvedic tradition comes from a disconnect between who we are and how we live.

What's Your *Dosha?*

So how do we work out what our *dosha* is?

Well, to do it properly, an Ayurvedic practitioner would conduct a physical exam and ask you questions to determine your mental and moral responses to different concepts and scenarios. They'd use these answers, and the exam, to work out which path to send you down. It's a skilled job – one that's been handed down from practitioner to practitioner over thousands of years. It requires a great deal of wisdom and many years of study. We can't hope to replicate that level of experience here, and I urge you, if this book sparks your curiosity, to seek out a practitioner for yourself.

In this book, however, in the absence of a true Ayurvedic practical exam, we're going to do a quick quiz. By the end of this chapter, you'll have a rough guide to the kind of personality type you might be in the Ayurvedic tradition, which will help you understand and navigate the rest of this book.

In the following chapters, we'll find various solutions and suggestions to resolve any places in our lives that feel unbalanced. Not all solutions will work for everyone, and not all suggestions will appeal to everyone – and that's where this quiz comes in. Some things will be recommended for some people, and not for others: it's as simple as that.

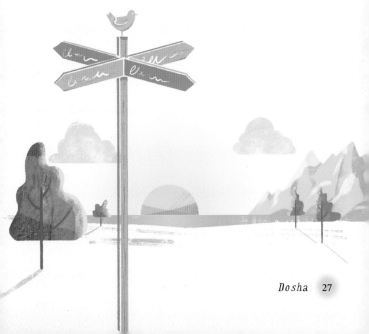

Taking the Quiz

Wherever something in this book depends on your *dosha*, ask yourself whether there might be something in this process you can learn from, something in it that can help you. Because something isn't working for you the way you're doing things right now, is it? Something is hard, and something is hurting. That's why you're here, right? You're here because, one way or another, things just aren't going the way you need them to, and the grooves of thought you've been caught in aren't helping.

Well, let's see whether we can find a better balance for you, where you are, right now, together.

Approach the book, the quiz and the question of your own balance with your most honest self and an open mind.

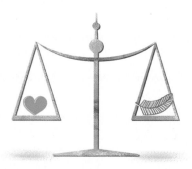

Find Your *Dosha*

Answer the following questions as honestly and fairly as you can. Grab a pen and paper and note down your answer for each question: A, B or C.

My body is…

A Curvy and heavy, with wide hips and shoulders.

B Medium build, fairly muscular without much effort and fairly well-proportioned.

C Slim and slight, with long limbs.

I tend to…

A Gain weight easily, unless I'm careful.

B Stay basically the same weight no matter what I do.

C Lose weight easily, unless I'm careful.

My skin is…

A Oily and soft.

B Combination and/or sensitive.

C Dry and rough.

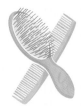

My hair is…

A Thick, shiny and glossy.

B Curly and/or dry.

C Straight and/or fine.

My body temperature runs…

A Too hot!

B Fine, mostly.

C Too cold!

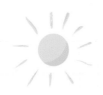

Given the choice, I would pick weather that is…

A Cool and dry.

B Warm and humid.

C Warm and dry.

My speech is…

A Slow, steady and considered.

B Sharp, concise and measured.

C Fast, and I talk a lot.

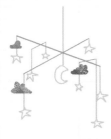

My sleep is…

A Good, but I can be lazy!

B Difficult at first, but then okay.

C Interrupted and prone to vivid dreams.

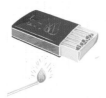

I'm drawn to…

A Earth.

B Air.

C Fire.

My main flaw is that I'm…

A Lazy.

B Judgmental.

C Spacey.

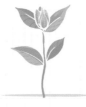

I'm great because I'm…

A Compassionate.

B Joyful.

C Determined.

The Results

Please remember that no judgment applies to these results; there's no value to being one *dosha* over another. Every body is a good body, and every way of being is a good way of being. What matters is being true to yourself.

Mostly As: You're a *kapha*! You're patient, grounded and caring. You're stable, reliable and great with people. You work well in a team. You sleep well. You have a real eye for beauty.

Mostly Bs: You're a *pitta*! You're an innovator with a Type-A personality, and you get stuff done. You know who you are, and you love it. You like being in control, but beware: sometimes this leads you to work too hard!

Mostly Cs: You're a *vata*! You're energetic, open-minded and quick to learn. You sometimes struggle with focus, and you're happiest outside, in nature.

This quiz is, of course, just a rough guide. The nature of *dosha* is such that it's very hard to determine on paper and for yourself. There are more detailed quizzes online. You may want to try a few before continuing with this book, to see how you feel.

2. Change

Agni

The common force among people of all three *doshas* is *agni*.

Agni is the essential pulse that unites all of us. It makes our bodies move and our cells divide. It turns food into energy and oxygen into carbon dioxide. It's the force that drives everything: it's the life force, essentially.

While the word *agni* literally translates as "fire", what it represents scientifically is metabolism. We've all heard of people described as having a "low" or "high" metabolism. But what does it really mean? Let's pause here for a quick science lesson.

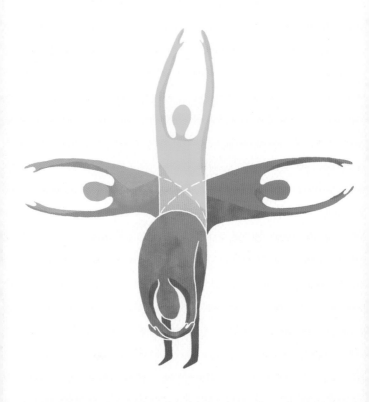

Understanding Metabolism

The word "metabolism" derives from the Greek word for "change". Metabolism is the process of continual change that happens within our bodies to keep us functioning: the breaking down (catabolism) and building up (anabolism) of cells. It describes all of the chemical processes inside the body that keep us alive, including digestion, breathing and healing.

These processes need energy, which is why we need to eat. They account (according to the UK's National Health Service) for between 40 and 70 per cent of our daily energy consumption. We call this your basal metabolic rate (BMR). A "slow" metabolism really just means a person has a low BMR. This BMR fluctuates according to your age, weight, build, gender and genetics. Your muscles and body fat, for instance, will change how "fast" your metabolism works.

It's incredible that these scientific ideas tally so exactly with something discovered five thousand years ago, but once we realize this, we can see how Ayurvedic medicine can work alongside Western science in order to help us live more fulfilling and balanced lives.

BMR and Calorie Calculators

There are many BMR calculators online, but a good rough formula on paper is:

- **Men:**
  BMR = (10 × weight in kg) + (6.25 × height in cm) – (5 × age in years) + 5

- **Women:**
  BMR = (10 × weight in kg) + (6.25 × height in cm) – (5 × age in years) – 161

Once you've worked out your BMR, you can apply it to the table opposite to calculate how many calories you need.

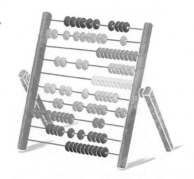

Lifestyle	Amount of exercise per week	Calorie Calculation
sedentary	little or no exercise	BMR × 1.2
lightly active	light exercise or sports on 1–3 days	BMR × 1.375
moderately active	moderate exercise or sports on 3–5 days	BMR × 1.55
very active	hard exercise or sports on 6–7 days	BMR × 1.725
extra active	very hard exercise or sports on 6–7 days and physical job	BMR × 1.9

Calculating your BMR and how many calories your body needs is, of course, the Western version of finding your *dosha*. As you can see, it's considerably less intuitive, and takes into account far fewer qualities than the Ayurvedic system. While at first glance, this system looks much more "scientific", the Ayurvedic approach actually gives us the freedom to think more clearly about the whole person, the whole self: not just our height and weight, but other things, too.

Ayurveda and the Modern World

It's important to note right now that Ayurveda should never replace modern medicine for serious illnesses, and should never be seen as a replacement for healthcare. There are no special prizes for skipping out on the benefits of modern science in the 21st century in order to more fully relish the joys of the 5th century BCE. Life in 5000 BCE was pretty difficult, and people suffered in ways we can't even imagine today. Furthermore, modern life brings stressors and health issues that ancient Ayurvedic practitioners could never have imagined.

What Ayurveda can do, however, is work with modern science to treat the body holistically: as that united, complete whole we talked about in Chapter 1. So where do we begin?

We begin by meeting ourselves where we are. We begin by acknowledging that perfection is impossible. An important part of Ayurveda is accepting who we are as a whole person: not aiming and striving to be somebody we're not, but simply being the best version of ourselves.

What Do *You* Need?

Take a few moments now to sit with yourself, and to carefully consider where you are and what you need.

How do you feel? Are you in any pain? Do you ache anywhere? Is anything feeling stiff? Notice where your body touches the floor or the chair. Notice how your wrists rest on your lap or at the table. Notice how this book feels in your hands. How do your toes feel? How about your ankles and your knees? Check in with your joints, one by one. Do you need to stretch? Do you need to move? Do you have any physical needs to attend to? Are your clothes uncomfortable? Do you need the bathroom? Are you tired or wired or hungry or thirsty? Check in with yourself.

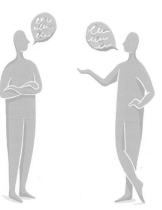

Over the next few pages, you'll find some suggestions to help you figure out what you need. But the most important thing is to listen to your body. You're the boss of you, and only you know what you need right now.

Hunger

Are you hungry? Are you too full? When did you last eat, and what was it? Did it satisfy you? Do you need to eat, or are you just bored? Is it really what you want? Do you want:

- A handful of almonds?

- A few raisins?

- A spoonful of nut butter?

- A couple of squares of dark chocolate?

- Nothing at all?

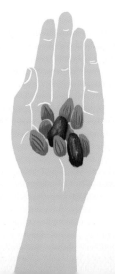

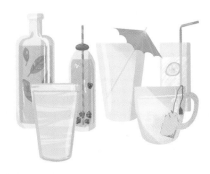

Thirst

Are you thirsty? When did you last drink, and what was it? Could you use a cool glass of water right now? (Spoiler: you could always benefit from a cool glass of water. Drink more water.)

Tiredness

How are your energy levels? Are you tired? Are you flagging at your desk? If you are, turn to page 89 for the Bellows Breath exercise, or throw yourself an emergency dance party: turn up your favourite song and dance for the full length of the tune – even if it's just in your chair. Dancing is guaranteed to lift your mood and bring energy back to your body. Be sure to move your fingers and toes, letting those good vibes flow through the full length of you.

Wiredness

Maybe you're feeling wired and can't calm down. Maybe you feel a bit all over the place, like there's just too much going on. Let's breathe together for a moment. Let's just notice our breath as it comes in and out of our lungs, not trying to change it yet, just noticing.

Sit with yourself for a minute, and then deepen the breath: breathe in for a count of four, hold for six, and then let it out for eight. In through the nose, out through the mouth. Picture your lungs filling and emptying, expanding and contracting. In, hold, out. In, hold, out. Do that until you've made a space within yourself to really focus on where you're going.

You may have noticed that a lot of this book is about noticing yourself. Maybe that feels obvious, but it's actually much harder than it looks. Bringing self-awareness into our daily lives is the point of pretty much all self-help advice. Once we bring ourselves into focus, it's much easier to make the changes we need to let ourselves be who we really are.

If your life is anything like mine, it's probably so busy you frequently lose sight of who you really are, and always were, and where you want to be. You need to declutter, mentally and physically. You need – deep breath here – to cleanse.

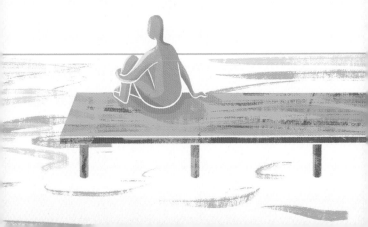

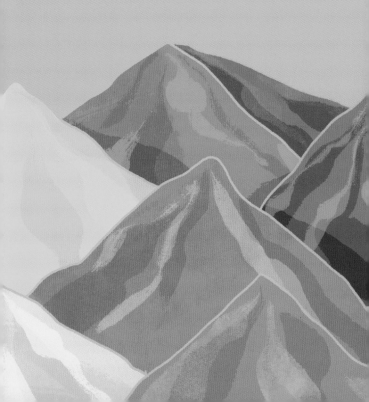

3. Cleanse

Panchakarma

The idea of a "cleanse" might be a difficult one. Cleanses are both fairly ubiquitous and fairly controversial – and, yet, sometimes, in some circumstances, they can work.

Ayurvedic cleanses are more properly known as *panchakarma*. Traditionally, an Ayurvedic practitioner would write a *panchakarma* tailored to fit your *dosha* and aligned to bring your *vikriti* and *prakriti* in line after a period of ill health or unease. A *panchakarma* reignites your *agni* when it might, perhaps, have become a little dim.

You can tell if your *agni* has gone out (or become dim) by considering the way you feel. Ask yourself:

- Are you fatigued?

- Are you irritable?

- Are you stiff and/or achy?

- Is your skin more oily than usual, or rougher and drier?

- Are you gaining or losing weight more quickly than you'd like?

- Do you feel just a little bit under the weather?

A key part of Ayurvedic medicine is learning to recognize your body's messages and warning signs. If we don't take care of these small aches and pains, things can quickly accumulate and escalate – and that's when the real problems start.

Ayurvedic cleanses are different to health-fad cleanses. They're not just about the physical process of the cleanse (the diet, exercise, and so on); they're also about what the cleanse can tell us about the rest of our life and how this can set us up for everything we want and need.

Ayurveda recommends doing a formal cleanse three times a year. The phrase "a formal cleanse" might seem off-putting, but don't worry. All we're going to do is use a set period of time to take stock of ourselves and what we're carrying with us. This period of time is usually divisible by three, and the cleanse in this book will last six days.

The six-day cleanse at the end of this chapter is inspired by Ayurvedic practices rather than being an authentic Ayurvedic cleanse. Ideally and traditionally, *panchakarma* should be dictated by healthcare and Ayurvedic professionals – and you should always consult a doctor before starting any cleanse, exercise programme or new regime.

The steps we're going to take to prepare for the cleanse should be accessible for everyone. However, if you feel compelled to try something more rigorous, check in with those healthcare professionals who know you best. Without knowing you, it could be dangerous for me to tell you how to change your diet, and that's not at all true to the Ayurvedic spirit. Remember, every body is different, and needs different care.

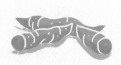 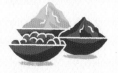

Preparing for the Cleanse

Before we begin the cleanse, we're going to review our consumption of alcohol, caffeine and sugar – and we're going to try to cut back where possible.

Now look, nowhere in this book will you find a condemnation of anyone for use of caffeine, sugar or alcohol. Ayurveda has space for all three, in moderation and in balance – and so does modern science. But these substances don't balance us, or restore us, or give us anything we're lacking. In fact, they can knock our *dosha* even further out of whack.

We need to be honest with ourselves. Is this really who we want to be? Is alcohol helping us to be the best we can be? Is sugar giving our bodies the best chance to be strong and capable? What will happen when the caffeine leaves our bloodstreams?

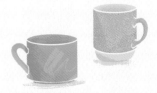

We often consume alcohol, caffeine or sugar to hide the fact that our basic needs aren't being met. Think back to that hierarchical pyramid in the introduction (see page 10). Do you turn to sugar because you're not eating the things your body needs? Do you turn to alcohol because you feel under-confident without it, or because you're too tired to bring your A-game without help? Do you turn to caffeine because you're lethargic? Are you using these substances to try and get by without the things you *really* need?

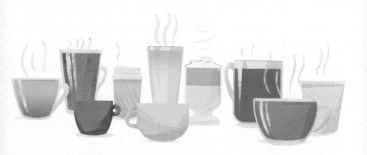

SELF-ASSESSMENT:

Alcohol

We all know that alcohol can cause serious damage to our bodies. Drinking too much puts pressure on our organs, especially the heart, which leads to high blood pressure, heart failure and strokes. This is in line with Ayurvedic teachings, again proving their remarkable prescience.

There are, of course, some benefits to drinking, which are acknowledged in both conventional and Ayurvedic wisdom. When taken correctly and in moderation, alcohol can not only help us to relax but also protect us against some forms of heart disease.

But what's moderation? A trained Ayurvedic practitioner may prescribe around 4–6 teaspoons with meals during a consultation. But I'm pretty sure that's not what we're going to find when we examine our own intakes. The only way to know what we're drinking is to note it down, and so before we begin our cleanse, we're going to take a preliminary week to assess where we are.

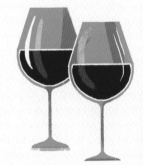

How Much Alcohol Do You Consume in a Week?

Use the space overleaf to keep a tally of your alcohol intake over the course of a week. We'll do it in points. Allocate the following points where applicable:

- one point for a half-pint (284ml/10fl oz) of low-strength beer (4 per cent) or a single measure of a spirit;

- two points for a medium glass of wine (175ml/6 fl oz) or double measure of a spirit);

- three points for one pint (568ml/20fl oz) of medium-strength beer (5 per cent).

It's a good idea to jot down a few notes about what prompted you to drink on those days as well as how you felt before drinking, how you felt while drinking and how you felt after drinking. Did you feel better or worse the next day?

WEEKLY ALCOHOL POINTS: ....

MONDAY

TUESDAY

WEDNESDAY

THURSDAY

FRIDAY

SATURDAY

SUNDAY

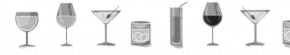

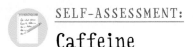

Caffeine

Caffeine is, perhaps, the most commonly used and abused psychoactive drug on the planet, and most of us don't even think twice about it. A famous study gave spiders various substances, and monitored the webs they spun as a result. On speed (Benzedrine), the spiders were able to keep their webs fairly steady. On marijuana, the webs looked pretty normal. But on caffeine? The webs were all over the place.

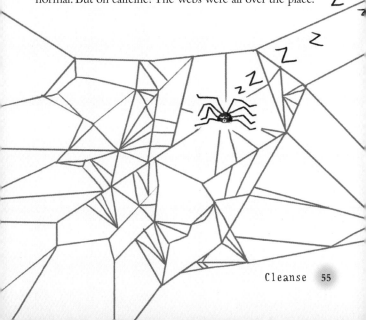

Part of the reason humans and animals need sleep is because of a chemical called adenosine. It builds up in our brains over the course of the waking day, and when it reaches a critical mass, we have to go to sleep. (This is vastly oversimplified, of course. Scientist Matthew Walker provides much more detail in his book *Why We Sleep*.)

Caffeine blocks the adenosine receptors in our brains – not the adenosine itself, but the receptors. This means we don't notice that the adenosine is amassing, or that we're getting tired, and that our bodies are – chemically – exhausted. When the caffeine wears off, the adenosine crashes into the receptors all at once – hence the phrase "caffeine crash".

When we don't have time to prepare ourselves for sleep, we can't respond to our bodies in the way they deserve and need. How can we listen to our bodies if we are deliberately silencing our impulses? (This also, of course, holds true for alcohol. When we dull our senses, we cut off the information we need to make smart choices for better balance.)

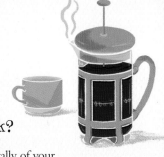

How Much Caffeine Do You Consume in a Week?

Use the space overleaf to keep a tally of your caffeine intake over the course of a week. Allocate:

- one point for a cup of tea;

- two points for a cup of coffee (at home);

- three points for a cup of coffee bought in a café or coffee shop.

These points are loosely based on an estimate of how much caffeine is in each of these drinks: about 75mg in a mug of tea, 100mg in a regular instant coffee and 140–200mg in a coffee from a café or coffee shop).

It's a good to jot down a few notes about what prompted you to turn to caffeine on those days, as well as how you felt before consuming the caffeine, how you felt directly afterward, and how you felt a few hours later. Did the effect last? Did it do what you needed it to do?

WEEKLY CAFFEINE POINTS: ....

MONDAY

TUESDAY

WEDNESDAY

THURSDAY

FRIDAY

SATURDAY

SUNDAY

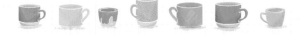

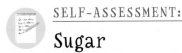
Sugar

Sugar is everyone's favourite demon right now. This makes sense, sort of: sugar has been linked to the obesity crisis, diabetes and high blood sugar. It's also, obviously, extremely bad for our teeth. Add that to the fact that tooth decay has been linked to gum trouble, and gum trouble to problems as severe and far-reaching as dementia, and it's certainly worth paying attention to how much sugar we consume.

But what does Ayurveda have to say on the subject? Well, this is where it gets interesting. Sweet is one of the "six tastes" of Ayurveda (something we'll explore in Chapter 4) and it's considered a necessary part of a balanced and healthy diet. However, we need to draw a distinction between the kinds of "sweet" food in Ayurvedic practice and the refined sugar that features in our diets today.

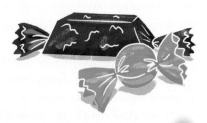

How Much Sugar Do You Consume in a Week?

It's hard to keep a tally of your sugar intake in the way we've done for caffeine and alcohol, so instead we're just going to keep an eye on it. Note when you add sugar to tea, or when you reach for a chocolate bar. Think about whether you're actually hungry, and whether feeding the sugar craving helped. What was it you from that sugar? Did it give you what you needed?

If you're scientifically minded, you may also want to jot down how many grams or ounces of sugar you find yourself eating per day. You can usually find this nutritional information on the back of the food packet or by using an app on your phone or laptop.

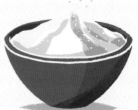

If this process is triggering or difficult for you, feel free to skip this step and turn instead to Chapter 4.

WEEKLY SUGAR INTAKE: ....

MONDAY

TUESDAY

WEDNESDAY

THURSDAY

FRIDAY

SATURDAY

SUNDAY

Time to Rebalance

If you're anything like me, the last few pages might have felt like quite a shock – both in terms of quantity and quality. What effects did you log? Were they positive or negative?

Who knew that we consumed so many things that have the power to hurt us? Who knew that we've been hurting ourselves in this way for so long? And now that we know, how do we stop? This is the point of a cleanse: to rid ourselves of the things we've been hanging on to for too long, and to free us of the things we've been doing without realizing it.

We need to let our *agni* shine. We need to undo the damage that's been building up every time we ignore a bad feeling and try to muffle it with unhealthy choices. We need to rebalance ourselves, and that's why this cleanse is helpful. It will give us a short period in which to be mindful and honest about who and what we are, and who and what we want to be.

It can be really difficult to realize how easily we reach for crutches like caffeine, alcohol and sugar, but you'll be amazed at how easy it can be to shake free of them.

Foods for the Cleanse

During the cleanse, you'll be eating very simply. It's called a "monodiet" because you're going to eat mostly the same things on rotation for the whole six days, which will give your body a chance to rest and reset. But don't worry, you won't go hungry!

You can modify the meals by checking in with your *dosha* recommendations (see pages 80–83). You might, for instance, add more chilli to balance out a *kapha* imbalance, or stir in some coconut milk for a troubled *pitta* personality. Listen to your body. What does it need?

There are three meals you will need to prepare during the cleanse: oats, kitchari and golden milk.

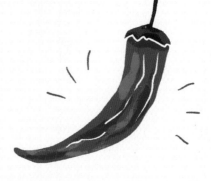

Oats

This is like a regular porridge, except it's made with ghee and boiling water. You can find detailed recipes for how to make it online and in Ayurvedic cookbooks, but here's the gist. Melt one tablespoon of ghee in a saucepan over a medium heat. Toss about four tablespoons of oats (steel-cut oats are best here, but any fine grains can also be substituted) into the melted ghee. Add a pinch of ground cinnamon and ginger (consider checking the requirements for your own *dosha* here), and stir again.

Cook for a few minutes over a low heat, then add a mug of boiling water (and perhaps some coconut milk). You can also add chopped dried fruit and nuts. (Dried apricots are great for a *vata*; apples for *pitta*; and any stewed fruit works well for *kapha*). Stir to a porridge-like consistency and cook for about ten minutes. Add a small pinch of salt, if your *dosha* allows, and enjoy.

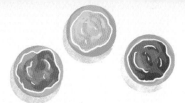

Kitchari

Recipes for kitchari can be found online and in many cookbooks. It's basically a rich, buttery dhal (a type of lentil stew), incorporating rice and fried spices. You should vary the spices according to your *dosha*, but the main ones are coriander, cumin, and mustard seeds. To make kitchari, place 250g (1 cup) yellow lentils (or similar pulses) and 100g (½ cup) rice in a saucepan of water over a medium heat. Cook for 20 minutes, or until soft. Meanwhile, melt a generous serving of ghee in a separate saucepan and quickly fry half a teaspoon of each spice. Drain the lentils and rice and stir in the spiced ghee. You could also add fresh ginger, fresh coriander and sesame seeds, if liked.

Golden Milk

Golden milk (*haldi doodh*), known in the West as a turmeric latte, has been a go-to home remedy in India for millennia. Whisk together a mug of almond milk (or other milk of your choice), one teaspoon of honey, a splash of vanilla extract, half a teaspoon of ground turmeric, a grating of nutmeg and a pinch of ground cinnamon and gently heat, frothing the whole time. Serve with a dusting of cinnamon.

The Six-Day Master Cleanse

The cleanse we're about to embark on is a six-day cleanse, but it's easy to adapt it for a twelve or even twenty-one day stretch. On each day of the cleanse, note down how you feel. Write down anything that comes to you, and anything that you'd like to follow up on in your life going forward. Allow yourself to feel your body. Let yourself feel your mind, your thoughts and your desires. Give yourself time to understand your needs. Listen to yourself. (And drink more water.)

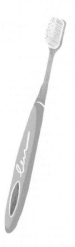

First Thing

Start each day with the 4-4 Breath exercise (see pages 86–88). Then, while brushing your teeth, take a moment to gently but firmly brush your tongue to remove any fuzziness that's built up overnight. (This might sound weird, but it's a key part of Ayurvedic practice. You can even buy special tongue scrapers for the task). Finally, fill a mug with warm boiled water. Swill some around your mouth after you've brushed your teeth, spit it out, then drink the rest.

Breakfast

On days one, five and six of the cleanse, start the day with oats (see page 64). On days two, three and four, start with kitchari (see page 65).

Morning Exercise

Whenever you can fit it into your day, do some gentle static exercise, like yoga. You'll find recommended yoga exercises that suit each *dosha* on pages 80–83. This needn't take long – perhaps 20 minutes.

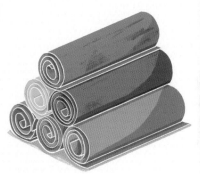

Lunch

For each day of the cleanse, eat kitchari for lunch. On days three, four, and five, consider adding an extra spoonful of ghee to your meal.

Afternoon Meditation

In the afternoon, make time to meditate. You'll find a breathing exercise for each *dosha* on pages 89–95. For each day of the cleanse, I'd like you to focus on a specific question:

Day 1: What brought me here?

Day 2: What matters to me?

Day 3: How do I feel physically?

Day 4: How do I feel mentally?

Day 5: How do I feel spiritually?

Day 6: Where do I want to go?

Take half an hour to get comfortable with the day's question. Grab a pen and paper so you can scribble down anything that occurs to you.

Sit cross-legged in whatever way feels best for you, with your hands resting on your knees, palms facing up. (If sitting cross-legged isn't possible for you, maybe just sit with your hands palm-up, as a symbol of openness.) A cushion can be useful here, too, to keep you comfortable and steady.

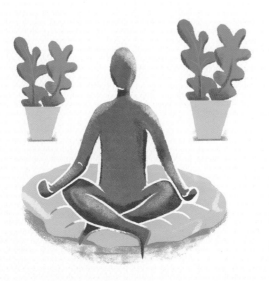

Start by noticing your breath. Follow the breath in and out, observing how it feels within you. Now, try to start emptying the mind – you're going to do that by counting to ten. Sounds easy, right? Well, maybe, but every time a thought comes into your head, you need to start again. Go back and start again, from one, every time you consciously notice anything, whether that's the numbers themselves or the sounds around you.

You're probably thinking this is impossible. And you're right. It's impossible for nearly everybody – but only if you think the goal is to get to ten. Which would be a ridiculous goal! Accept your thoughts, accept them with joy, and then turn your attention back each time to the breath.

The purpose of this exercise is to prepare your mind to consider what you're doing with it. You're learning to focus your attention on yourself. Do this for ten minutes, and then consider the question of the day. Consider the question in both the broadest and smallest senses possible, from the most mundane to the perfectly divine. Jot down any feelings or thoughts that come to you as you meditate.

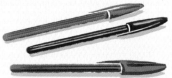

Dinner

Dinner is more kitchari (there's that monodiet again!),
followed by golden milk (see page 65). It's common
knowledge that a warm, milky drink aids sleep, and turmeric
aids all kinds of *agni* within the body.

Before Bed

Take a moment to consider how you feel and make a few
notes. Then end the day with the 4-4 Breath (see pages
86–88). Breathe deeply. Breathe well. How do you feel?
How is this diet working for you? How much energy do
you have? How are you? Where are you? What do you want?
What do you need?

Try to get plenty of rest. Try to stay off your screen and try
not to worry too much about whether you're doing this
whole cleanse thing "right". I promise you, whatever
modifications you're making are completely fine. Whatever
you're doing, however you're showing up for yourself, is fine.

4. Nourish, Move, Glow

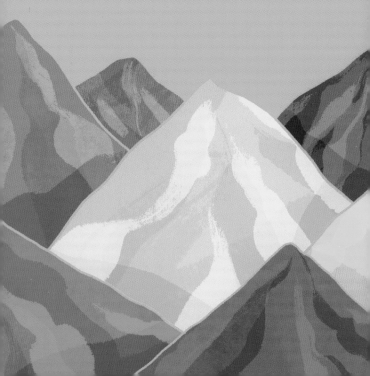

Listen to Your Body

Ayurveda is about accepting yourself as a united being: mind, body and soul in one. Too often with self-help, we drift away from the physical and into the emotional, focusing on metaphorical feelings, and ignoring the warning signs of the body. If you take one thing from this book, let it be this: we are our own best teachers. Every day, our bodies give us cues and signals as to what we want and need. They prompt us to eat when we are hungry, to drink when we are thirsty, to move, to rest, to sleep. Our bodies are perfectly calibrated calculators, miraculously and wonderfully made to compute the nutrients we need.

In this chapter, we're going to look at the best ways to move and nourish our bodies. We'll be concentrating on one *dosha* at a time – but remember that we can all feel different elements of the *doshas*, no matter our *prakriti*. That's why we need to start listening to ourselves; that's why we need to keep asking ourselves what we need, and who we are, and what we want.

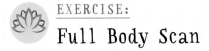

EXERCISE:

Full Body Scan

This exercise comes, at least in part, from a mindfulness exercise called a "body scan".

1 Lie comfortably wherever suits you – on a yoga mat, bed or sofa.

2 Breathe deeply. Don't modulate your breath, here. It belongs to you, and it's sustained you for your whole life. Notice your breath; acknowledge its presence. Acknowledge how it feels in your mouth and in your lungs and in your belly. Acknowledge how you feel as the breath moves in and out of your lungs. Respect your breath as it is, and meet yourself exactly where you are. (This is going to be important in the exercises that follow. We must meet ourselves where we are, at our appropriate edge. We must not try to be more. We must not settle for less. This is it. We are where we are. We are who we are.) Breathe deeply, and pay attention.

3 How does your breath feel in your throat, your chest, your lungs, your diaphragm? Really notice your breath, your pulse, the way your body rests against itself and the surface of your yoga mat, sofa or bed.

4 How do you feel? How do you feel about doing this exercise? Do you feel restless or stupid? Is there part of your mind that thinks you ought to be doing something else right now? Accept any thoughts that come into your mind: as in Zen practice, feel grateful both to have the thought and to have noticed it.

5 Bring your attention to the toes on your feet. Start with your big toes. What do your big toes feel like? Are they touching anything? Can you feel your socks? Focus, then draw your attention to the next toe along. And the next. Each toe in turn deserves your attention. Move your attention up through the soles of the feet, the arches, the heels, the ankles.

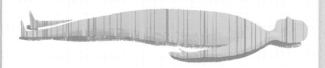

6 Run your attention up your calves and to your knees. Notice any pain or tension, any sensation or lack of sensation. Notice how your skin feels against your clothing. Bring your attention very slowly up your legs to your thighs and hips. Breathe.

7 Feel the breath move through your body. Let your attention, with the breath, move from your feet into your legs, and from your legs into your torso, noticing any sensations or emotions. Breathe.

8 Let your attention move into your arms and down to your elbows, your hands, your fingers and fingertips. Breathe deeply. Notice anything, notice everything, notice nothing.

9 Breathe in, breathe out. Slowly move your attention back up your arms and into your neck, your shoulders, your throat and chin and cheeks, your mouth, nose, eyes, ears and scalp. Each part of you is valid. Breathe.

10 When you're ready, open your eyes. Give yourself a moment or two to notice the world around you: the light, the atmosphere.

Now, listen to the messages of your body. Are you hungry? Are you thirsty? Are you in discomfort or pain? Do you need anything? Do you need to stretch, or move, or eat, or drink? Listen to your body, your clever, wise, dependable body. Recognize the signals it sends.

We do this exercise because it forces us to pay attention to what's really there, and nothing else. By taking this time for ourselves, we begin to see who we are, and who we can be. It will help us restore what is lost, mend what is damaged and balance what has become unbalanced.

Mind and Body in Harmony

We can't hope to be at our best mentally unless we are also at our best physically. How can we find balance unless the two are in harmony? In order to find mental clarity we need to nourish our bodies with food, water and exercise.

We can't rest well unless we are tired; we don't tire unless we move; we can't move if we don't eat the right foods, drink the right beverages and of course, rest well in turn (and so the natural cycle comes round again). It's always about balance. As we rest, so must we move: a little from column A, a little from column B.

Ayurveda recommends exercising at 50 per cent of our capacity: just enough to raise a light sweat, but no more. We don't need to push ourselves to our outer limits. You've heard people say "no pain, no gain"? Well, that's just not true. Small movements can make vast differences: from a tiny acorn, a mighty oak can grow. One of the most beautiful systems of small movements is yoga, and it has been a part of Ayurvedic practice for millennia. It's even argued by some that Patanjali, the founding father of yoga, and Charaka, the founding father of Ayurveda, are one and the same.

Over the next few pages, we'll look at the yoga exercises and foods best suited to each *dosha*.

What Does Your Body Need to Be Balanced?

There are six tastes in Ayurvedic medicine – sweet, sour, salty, pungent, bitter and astringent – and each *dosha* has them naturally in different measures. We need to eat a diet that reflects what we lack, in order to become our most balanced selves. Some things, like ginger, for instance are good for everyone; some things, like meat, should be eaten in moderation. And, of course, we can all benefit from drinking more water.

While traditionally some foods have been seen as "bad" or "good" for each *dosha* (and you'll find some examples on the following pages), the approach we've adopted in this book is much more about listening to your body. What do you really want? What do you really need? What would help you feel balanced today?

Kapha

Nature: Oily, soft, cold, moist, dull, static, smooth, heavy.

Element: Earth.

Preferred tastes: Sweet, sour, salty.

Digestion: Slow, regular, good appetite.

People with *kapha* systems need to make lifestyle choices that are by nature hot, dry, clear and sharp; they need to choose more active lifestyles than other *doshas*; and they need more exercise. They need to eat to be stimulated and warmed, and they need to move vigorously and regularly to keep themselves active.

Recommended tastes: Salty, pungent, bitter.

Recommended foods: Barley, rye, apples, seeds, beans, spices, greens, garlic, buttermilk.

Foods to try to stay away from: Fat, oil, cooked honey, raw dairy, salt, olives, oats.

Recommended yoga poses: Sun Salutation, Warrior II (see page 83).

Pitta

Nature: Sharp, liquid, light, spreading, hot.

Element: Fire.

Preferred tastes: Salty, sour, pungent.

Digestion: Very good, with a good appetite and strong metabolism.

Exercise is naturally very good for encouraging *pitta,* so people with a *pitta* system need to try not to outdo themselves! They need rough, cold, heavy, static experiences to counteract their natural tendency for fast, liquid movements; and they need to find a balance between their more competitive instincts and the need to relax. The recommended yoga poses below help *pitta* people to find stillness. It's important that *pitta* people don't overheat.

Recommended tastes: Dry, astringent, bitter, sweet.

Recommended foods: Coriander, mint, coconuts, pomegranates, vegetables, rice.

Foods to try to stay away from: Spicy foods, garlic, tomatoes, radishes, chillies, sour dairy.

Recommended yoga poses: Shoulder Stand, Cobra (see page 83).

Vata

Nature: Dry, subtle, light, rough, clear, active, cold, mobile.

Element: Air.

Preferred tastes: Pungent, bitter, astringent.

Digestion: Irregular and erratic, easily aggravated.

Vata is the most delicate *dosha*, and the most easily troubled; the yoga poses recommended below are steadying, smooth, sticky poses that help people with *vata* systems connect with the earth in a meaningful and purposeful way. *Vata* people need to find stability and connection, and the recommended foods are all heavy and soft. The foods should be fluid, flexible and steadying to balance *vata* people, who tend to have airy and flighty natures.

Recommended tastes: Salty, sour, sweet.

Recommended foods: Warm food, dairy (butter on everything), rice, wheat, avocados, cream.

Foods to try to stay away from: Spices, chillies and other spicy foods.

Recommended yoga poses: Forward Fold, Child's Pose (see opposite).

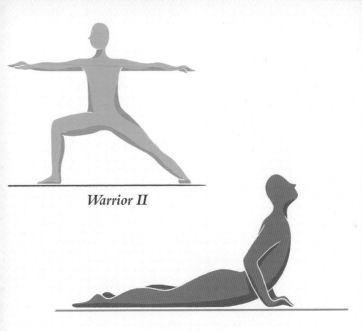

Warrior II

Cobra

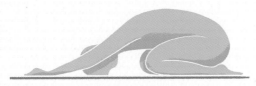

Child's Pose

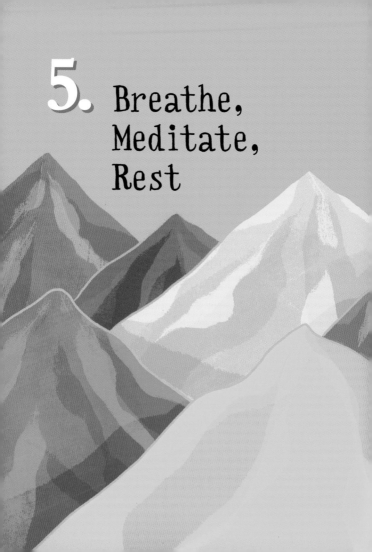

5. Breathe, Meditate, Rest

Breathing and Meditation

You might think breathing should be intuitive, and in some ways, you're right. We're all breathing, all the time, and we've been doing fine so far, or we wouldn't still be here. Well, sure. But this book isn't about being "fine". It's about being the best self we can be, and how we breathe can help us do that.

Pranayama, the ancient art of breathing, is deeply and profoundly connected to meditation: it's the act of mindfully belonging to the moment in which you live. This meditative breathing is how we learn to rest, and how we find the peace we need to restore and rejuvenate our tired minds.

In this chapter, you'll find breathing exercises for each *dosha*. Of course, you're not limited only to the exercises recommended for your *dosha*. It's just a question of balance. Choose what feels right for you. Don't push yourself too hard, or force yourself into any attitude that feels like it's going against your wellbeing. You know you best.

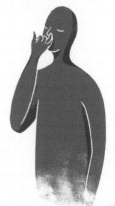

The 4-4 Breath

Let's start with an exercise we can do together, right now, wherever we are.

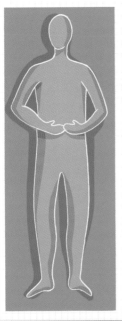

1 Sit or lie down somewhere you won't be disturbed for ten minutes. Make sure you're comfortable, and that you can hold this posture easily. Relax, and bring your hands up to your ribcage. Your palms should sit just above the base of your ribcage.

2 Breathe in and out normally, and try to notice your breath. Follow the thread of your breath as it moves into your lungs and diaphragm, and up out through your throat, mouth and nose.

3 When you feel comfortable, try to start evening
out your breath – breathe in through the nose,
and then out through the mouth. Breathe in for a
count of four, and out for four. Count it in your
head: in, two, three, four; out, two, three, four. Try to
keep the breaths steady. Let the pressure of the air
be the same on each beat. Focus on your breath.

4 You'll be able to feel if you're doing this right
because your ribs will move under your palms,
and your shoulders will rise and fall in an even
pattern. Think of how you breathe when you sleep:
steady, regular, uninterrupted.

5 Picture yourself breathing *into* your palms as they
lie on your ribs. Are your palms moving? Can
you make them move by breathing into the four
corners of your lungs? Let the air fill your body
deeply, and then empty it all out. Keep counting
the steady beats of your breathing. If you need to
slow the counting down or speed it up, that's okay.
Focus on the breath at hand.

6 Take ten minutes to really get into this exercise. If a thought enters your mind, acknowledge it (do so joyfully – you haven't failed, it's okay to have other thoughts), then return your conscious thought to the breath.

7 When you're ready, ask yourself:

- How does the breath feel in my mouth and my nose? How about in my chest and my lungs?

- How does my body feel when I breathe in? How does it feel when I breathe out? How do I feel for having spent this time with my breath?

Fantastic work. It's always a good idea to begin with a breath exercise designed to take you to a place of calm. This will help us bring our full attention to the work of rebalancing our bodies in the following exercises.

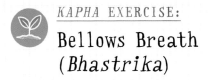

KAPHA EXERCISE:

Bellows Breath (*Bhastrika*)

Kapha people tend to be slow, and sometimes lazy or sluggish. They need to make themselves move in order to counterbalance their natural slowness. While we do this breathing exercise, which is designed to bring a little fire into our bellies, it's useful for *Kaphas* to try and run through the yogic moves mentioned on page 83.

1 Stand up, with your arms resting by your sides. Your back should be as straight as you can make it. Your hips should be over your feet and your shoulders in line with your hips. Your head should be directly over your heart, and your heart over your pelvis. Can you bring your shoulder blades together?

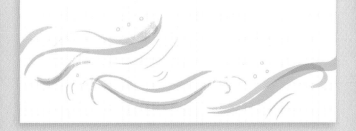

2 Breathe for a few moments in the 4–4 pattern we practised earlier (see pages 86–88), and then we'll start to move.

3 Inhale forcefully through your nostrils for a count of four, bringing the air down to your belly, and swinging your arms up above your head as you do so (keep them straight!).

4 Exhale, equally forcefully, for a count of four again, lowering your arms back down by your sides.

5 Repeat for two minutes, focusing entirely on your breath, the movement of the air in and out of your belly, and the movement of your arms through the air.

Cooling Breaths (*Sitali* and *Sitkari* Pranayama)

Pitta is the fire *dosha*, with characteristics including hot, oily, light and sharp, which can make us become angry or frustrated. These two breathing exercises are designed to cool us down and make us think about our actions.

Sitkari

This exercise is best undertaken after you've done the 4–4 Breath (see pages 86–88).

1 Get your breath regular and even. Become comfortable with yourself and close your eyes.

2 Press your teeth together and draw your lips back as far as they will comfortably go – imagine an angry cartoon cat. This may seem a little weird, but it has a purpose. You should be able to feel the air cool against your gums, and that cooling effect is what this is all about.

3 Keeping your breathing steady, inhale through the gaps in the teeth for a count of four. Listen to the hiss of air, cooling through your mouth and throat, down into your lungs and belly.

4 Relax your lips, close your mouth, and exhale through the nose. Repeat for at least 20 breaths.

Sitali

You need to be able to roll your tongue for this exercise. If you can't do it, don't worry; instead try picturing a green leaf uncurling or the beak of a bird – these images can help you focus your mind on what you want your tongue to do.

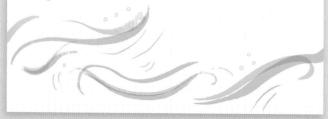

1 Sit comfortably. Visualize your spine as a straight line (maybe imagine a taut piece of string connecting the crown of your head with your pelvis). Bring your attention to your breath; as ever, keep that 4-4 even regularity. Let it touch all four corners of the lungs.

2 Bring the air in through the mouth, and out through the nose. Open your mouth into an O-shape. If you can, poke out your tongue, and curl it into a U-shape. (If you can't, picture a curling leaf or a bird's beak.) Now, inhale through your curled-up tongue, as if it were a drinking straw. Retract your tongue, close your mouth and exhale through the nose.

3 Repeat for eight breaths. Give yourself eight regular deep breaths and then repeat the cooling breath eight times.

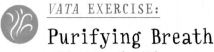

VATA EXERCISE:

Purifying Breath (*Nadi Shodhana*)

Vata's elemental characteristics are dry, cold, light, rough and mobile, which can make *vata* people anxious or nervous. This purifying breath will help us to clear our minds and find peace. It's great for when you're feeling panicky or overwhelmed.

1 Sit comfortably, with a straight, tall back. Visualize your spine as a straight line (maybe imagine a taut piece of string connecting the crown of your head with your pelvis).

2 Put the index finger and middle finger of your right hand on your forehead, above your nose. Cover your right nostril with your thumb and close your mouth.

3 Breathe in, for a count of eight, through your open left nostril. Then, cover your left nostril with your fourth finger and release your thumb. Breathe out, for the same count of eight, through your right nostril.

4 Keeping your left nostril closed, breathe in through the same open right nostril, for a count of eight.

5 Close your right nostril with your thumb and release your fourth finger. Breathe out, for the same count of eight, through your open left nostril.

6 Repeat for 12 rounds.

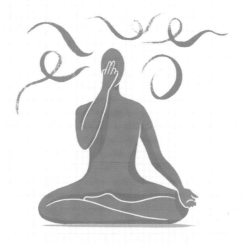

What Have You Learned?

One you've finished the breathing exercise for your *dosha*, ask yourself:

- How does the breath feel in my mouth and nose? How about in my chest? My lungs?

- How does my body feel when I breathe in? How does it feel when I breathe out?

- How do I feel for having spent this time with my breath?

- How do I feel for having spent this time with myself?

The last question is, perhaps, the central question of this book. How do I feel having spent this time with myself? What have I learned? What can I take from this experience? How can I become more balanced?

Let's come together one last time to reflect on what we've learned. Lie down and mindfully consider the ways we can take the lessons from this book into our lives. We need to listen to our bodies; eat more intuitively; find the rest we need; leave behind the things that swing us out of balance; and come to a deeper sense of being the best version of ourselves that we can be.